Surviving OSHA
How to Avoid, Manage, and Respond to Healthcare Inspections

Kenneth S. Weinberg, BA, MSc, PhD

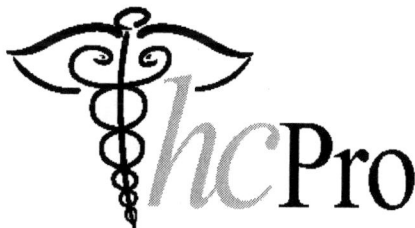

*hc*Pro

Surviving OSHA: How to Avoid, Manage, and Respond to Healthcare Inspections is published by HCPro, Inc.

Copyright 2004 by HCPro, Inc.

ISBN 1-57839-465-1

HCPro, Inc., provides information resources for the healthcare industry.

HCPro, Inc., is not affiliated in any way with the Joint Commission on Accreditation of Healthcare Organizations, which owns the JCAHO trademark.

Kenneth S. Weinberg, BA, MSc, PhD, Author
Steven A. MacAuthur, Contributing Editor
Judith Kelliher, Senior Managing Editor
Rebecca Silverman, Copy Editor
Mike Michaud, Layout Artist
Alison Forman, Proofreader
Jackie Diehl Singer, Graphic Artist
Tom Philbrook, Cover Designer
Jean St. Pierre, Creative Director
Bob Croce, Group Publisher
Suzanne Perney, Publisher

Advice given is general. Readers should consult professional counsel for specific legal, ethical, or clinical questions. Arrangements can be made for quantity discounts.

For more information, contact:

HCPro, Inc.
P.O. Box 1168
Marblehead, MA 01945
Telephone: 800/650-6787 or 781/639-1872
Fax: 800/639-8511 or 781/639-2982
E-mail: *customerservice@hcpro.com*

Visit HCPro at its World Wide Web site
www.hcpro.com

10/2004
20134

Contents

About the author

Kenneth S. Weinberg, BA, MSc, PhD

Kenneth S. Weinberg, BA, MSc, PhD, is president and principal consultant of Safdoc Systems, LLC, based in Stoughton, MA. Safdoc specializes in environmental health and safety and toxicology.

His extensive experience in healthcare and healthcare safety includes serving as director of safety at Massachusetts General Hospital in Boston for more than 10 years.

Weinberg is a professional member of the American Society of Safety Engineers (ASSE) and for two years was the administrator of its HealthCare Division. In addition, he is listed in the National Registry of Safety Professionals and is a registered professional industrial hygienist. He is a Certified Toxics Use Reduction Planner for general practice. In 2001, the Healthcare Specialty Practice of ASSE at its annual Professional Development Conference named Weinberg Safety Professional of the Year.

Weinberg's educational background and training includes a bachelor's degree in biology from Boston University, a master's degree in environmental health and radiation health physics from the University of Pittsburgh Graduate School of Public Health, and a doctorate in biochemistry and pathology from Boston University Graduate School's Division of Medical and Dental Sciences.

In addition to his consulting work, Weinberg teaches, writes articles for professional journals, and speaks during conferences and seminars around the country. He is an editor of several national safety publications, and has contributed chapters for books on health and safety.

Weinberg has authored three books, the first and second editions of *The Hospital Safety Director's Handbook* and *Indoor Air Quality During Construction: A Guide to Best Engineering Practices and Regulatory Compliance*, all published by HCPro.

Dedication

This book is dedicated to my constant companion and inspiration, Natalie.

Stoughton, MA
September 1, 2004

Introduction

The influence of OSHA on worker safety has not disappeared, though it has changed somewhat from a regulatory perspective. Even without the promulgation of new regulations and despite the withdrawal of some regulations, most notably the transition of the ergonomics standard to ergonomics "guidelines," you need only look as far as the recent upswing in enforcement activities relative to health-care and the tuberculosis respirator standard to determine that OSHA remains a strong and viable agency.

OSHA's efforts at providing more assistance to employers in reducing worker injuries and illness, as well as safety and hazard reduction compliance in general, have not resulted in reduced enforcement of existing standards. In the absence of specific standards, as in the case of ergonomics, an inspector may still conduct a survey of your healthcare facility. When a facility can neither demonstrate compli-ance, nor even a good-faith effort to comply with a standard or a guideline that is not a regulatory standard, an OSHA inspector still has the power to issue cita-tions—and even fine you—under its General Duty Clause (GDC). The GDC reflects the provisions of Section 5 of the OSHA Act of 1970. It requires employ-ers (and employees) to work as a "general duty" to ensure a safe workplace. Section 5 duties set the following requirements for both employers and employees:

Each employer:
- Shall furnish to each of his employees employment and a place of employ-ment which are free from recognized hazards that are causing or are likely to cause death or serious physical harm to his employees

- Shall comply with occupational safety and health standards promulgated under this Act

- Shall comply with occupational safety and health standards promulgated under this Act, which are applicable to his own actions and conduct

Because the nature of the OSHA standard, as underscored by the GDC, is to help employers understand that their obligation is to provide employees with a "safe and healthful" workplace that is free from recognized "safety and health" hazards, inspectors have the authority to issue citations and fines under these circumstances.

OSHA may interact with your organization in several different ways, but will work primarily through a survey or an on-site inspection of your facility. A survey (which is conducted by OSHA on an annual basis—usually to earmarked industries) is basically a request by OSHA for the provision of facility-specific illness and injury information for the purposes of data collection pursuant to Standard 1904.41, annual OSHA injury and illness reporting of 10 or more employers.

An on-site inspection, on the other hand, is a rather more invasive proposition, though there are certainly some predictors that can be used to identify the likelihood of your organization being identified for OSHA inspection. We'll look at these predictors more closely in Chapter 3, Events that prompt OSHA action.

If OSHA conducts an inspection in your facility and finds evidence of violations, the penalties may range from fines to ongoing surveillance. Negative OSHA inspections can be embarrassing to your facility and cost thousands of dollars in fines. OSHA violations can even lead to a loss of revenue, as potential clients, such as pharmaceutical firms who underwrite research activities, and patients are less inclined to enter a facility where documented problems were made public.

This text covers a variety of topics, all designed to assist you in avoiding these costly and embarrassing issues by first taking steps to reduce the likelihood of an OSHA inspection. If you undergo an inspection, the text also discusses the proper ways to treat the inspector. If you are cited, the text provides advice on handling and responding to the results of the inspection, citations, and fines.

Chapter

1

OSHA oversight

OSHA oversight

Those who work in healthcare, particularly administrators, environmental health and safety professionals, and attorneys, almost unanimously agree that healthcare organizations are among the most scrutinized and regulated businesses in the United States. There are many reasons for this intense oversight, including a desire to keep healthcare costs in check while providing quality care and safety for patients.

A wide array of regulations governs healthcare organizations. The discussion in this chapter will be limited to those requirements that OSHA promulgates and enforces. However, there are other regulatory issues that concern many hospital administrators and safety professionals. One of these issues centers on environmental safety outside the facility, which the Environmental Protection Agency (EPA) oversees.

Through the late 1980s, OSHA and the EPA enforced their regulations primarily in industry sectors, virtually overlooking the healthcare industry. For all intents and purposes, regulatory agencies did not even consider hospitals, nursing homes, or rehabilitation facilities as being significant contributors to worker injury and illness or to environmental pollution. However, in the late 1980s and early 1990s, these stances changed.

A number of factors prompted this shift, including the regulatory scrutiny that came with the passage of OSHA's Hazard Communication standard. This standard opened the doors for regulators such as OSHA to look more closely at the practices of healthcare facilities and their management of the use of hazardous chemicals. Soon after the passage of the Hazard Communication standard, a flurry of events prompted even further regulatory awareness of healthcare facilities, especially as the procedures relating to AIDS and other bloodborne pathogens, the use of latex gloves and its negative effect on health, and questions regarding the disposal of infectious waste, demonstrated the potentially deleterious impact of various practices in healthcare that could affect not only hospital employees, but also workers in the waste disposal industry and the general public.

At the same time, the rising costs of infectious waste disposal led to an increase in medical waste incinerators, resulting in more scrutiny of the hazards these incinerators generated. Regulators became and continue to be concerned with, among other issues, emissions of dioxins from the burning of plastics, and the release of a variety of toxic metals, such as zinc and mercury, into the waste water system. As a direct result of these concerns, the government soon identified hospitals and dental offices as major contributors to environmental mercury pollution. Regulators from all areas of health and safety began to focus on healthcare's contributions to illness and injury among employees and the larger community.

Now healthcare organizations are considered participants in both regulatory arenas: occupational injury and illness, and the effects that workplaces have on the environment.

Handling hazardous chemicals

One of the first regulations that affected healthcare institutions involved the handling of hazardous workplace chemicals, but hospital administrators felt they should be exempt from this regulation. Healthcare administrators believed that they had no or very few hazardous chemicals on site, and that those chemicals that were present were in such small quantities they were not of any consequence to employees or to the people who lived in the surrounding community.

As such, when the OSHA Hazard Communication standard first passed in 1986, hospitals believed this standard applied to other businesses. Of course, as we now know, hospitals lost the argument, primarily because the regulators and those representing healthcare workers strongly believed that the nature, volume, and types of hazardous materials that hospital workers handled and used were not fully understood and, that as a result, the hazards these materials posed were underestimated. The institution of this new law would help, in the opinion of those subject to the regulations to highlight the nature of the hazards that healthcare workers faced and thus would help reduce the number of injuries and illnesses that healthcare workers endured due to deficient education and training relative to their exposure to hazardous materials and waste.

The reporting and tallying (inventorying) of hazardous chemicals, as a function of managing the associated risks to employees, became a key responsibility of health-care safety professionals. Review of the hazard communication program became an important part of OSHA's newly emerging regulatory oversight of hospitals. What's more, this particular regulation continues to be at the forefront of OSHA inspections and compliance activities conducted in healthcare facilities, as well as in other industries.

Virtually every OSHA inspector who walks through the front door of a hospital, nursing home, or long-term care facility to conduct an inspection will review the hospital's hazard communication program. The interesting fact is that the "HazCom" standard, as it is called, remains one of the top five cited standards by inspectors, even in healthcare. In 2003, the HazCom standard was the most frequently cited standard in all industries, accounting for $1.3 million in fines and 7,009 violations. In healthcare, only the bloodborne pathogen standard was cited more often than the Hazard Communication standard, yet the latter still accounted for more than $6,000 in penalties between October 2002 and October 2003.

Bloodborne Pathogen standard

Other OSHA regulations have significantly impacted the healthcare industry. An example is the Bloodborne Pathogen (BBP) standard, which was enacted in response to the probability that healthcare workers in a variety of settings, as well as those who work as emergency responders, will face exposure to BBPs during their regular work duties. Violation of the BBP standard has become the number one violation OSHA inspectors cite. Going hand in hand with this regulation is an amendment to OSHA's Bloodborne Pathogen standard—the Health Care Worker Needle Stick Prevention Act of 1999—which was designed to reduce sharps injuries and record and track sharps exposures. The act clearly outlines the proactive role mandated of healthcare employers; sharps safety programs must reflect an ongoing evaluation of the risks associated with the use of sharps in healthcare.

The Health Care Worker Needle Stick Prevention Act passed following the collection of 10 years of data showing that the top injuries related to BBPs were due to needlesticks and sharps mishaps. This act also called for OSHA to update and revamp its BBP requirements by adding new definitions, including what constitutes a safe needle device. In addition, the updated standard required employers to include frontline staff in the decision-making processes surrounding the selection of new, safe needle devices as well as the ongoing review of devices currently in use.

Respiratory protection and tuberculosis

One of the more challenging, and perhaps unexpected, regulations applied to healthcare is OSHA's Respiratory Protection standard. A great deal of movement and change has occurred within the handling of this standard over the past decade. Part of this change results directly from the recognition that healthcare workers must wear respirators for protection against patients infected with tuberculosis (TB). In the early 1990s, multidrug resistant forms of TB were on the rise among several populations. In addition, strains of TB were found to be resistant to the usual medical treatments, especially among immunocompromised patients already suffering from AIDS.

The increase in TB cases in several United States cities caught both regulators and healthcare professionals off guard, particularly since the occurrence of TB cases in the United States, in general, had been considered almost nonexistent. As a result, no real guidelines existed at the time for the types of precautions to take when dealing with TB-infected individuals, except for the normal recommendations of using a surgical mask and gown.

The first response to this new TB epidemic came from the Centers for Disease Control and Prevention (CDC), which put forth guidelines as early as 1992 for worker protection against TB infection, including the use of high-efficiency particulate air respirators. Hospitals and other healthcare providers did not know how to best respond to the recommendations from the CDC and, in particular, how to ensure that care providers were properly equipped with respirators.

As healthcare organizations were sorting out these issues, OSHA stepped in and proposed a TB standard that at first seemed to be on the fast track for passage. Part of OSHA's proposal resulted in the enactment of a respirator standard specifically aimed at healthcare workers to guide and assist them in the proper selection and use of respirators (known as "N95" respirators) when exposed to TB patients.

After almost seven years on the table, OSHA withdrew its proposed TB standard, stating that because the proposal was so close to the CDC guidelines, and hospitals and all other healthcare providers were already following the CDC guidelines, there was no need to duplicate the effort. The existing TB respirator standard (29 CFR 1910.139) was also withdrawn and referred back to the existing standard for respirator use and selection (29 CFR 1910.134). However, over the course of the existence of the proposed standard, OSHA performed inspections, responded to complaints, and issued citations and penalties to healthcare organizations, using the requirements of the standard as a compliance guide. OSHA cited facilities for failure to comply with the TB respirator standard or other elements of worker TB protection requirements using the general duty clause (GDC) of the OSHA standard as its basis for citations. As such, citations were issued under the GDC because the OSHA TB standard did not actually exist as a law.

The GDC, which states at least in part that employers must provide their employees with a workplace free from recognized hazards, is at the heart of the requirement (and sensible practice) that employers conduct a complete survey of their facilities in order to identify such hazards. TB is one such hazard in healthcare, so logically a facility could be cited for violating the GDC if it does not offer employees appropriate protection from this hazard. Some cynics state that it is for this reason that safety officers or other hospital employees do not record the hazards they observe when conducting surveys of their facilities, thus avoiding inclusion of these hazards as part of the list of recognized hazards of the facility. Therefore, OSHA compliance officers cannot use these hazards as evidence for a citation.

This is flawed logic, from which no good can come. Certainly, the hazards of healthcare as an industry are well documented in a variety of places by a number of observers. The result is that unless there is a specific reason that a facility is exempt from a hazard requirement, such as the respiratory protection standard, and the facility can document the reasons why it is exempt, safety officers and administrators should spend their time documenting the issues as they exist in the facility and the measures they are taking to address and correct them.

Ergonomics guidelines

More recently, OSHA enacted ergonomics legislation aimed at a number of industries, with both nursing homes and hospitals high on the list. Congress passed this legislation and then-departing President Clinton signed it into law. The regulation was controversial among industry and regulatory observers. Both sides expressed a number of opinions on the regulation concerning the appropriateness of its content, the way it was enacted, and the impact that it would have on healthcare and other industries. As a result, the incoming Bush Administration quickly repealed the regulation.

In its place, OSHA chief John L. Henshaw, along with federal Secretary of Labor Elaine L. Chao, developed a creative replacement for the regulation: voluntary ergonomics guidelines. These guidelines were the result of discussions held among numerous stakeholders, such as labor organizations, healthcare workers, and ergonomics experts. The resulting document was a compilation of recommendations and ergonomic best practices that, it was believed, could reduce the number of musculoskeletal injuries in healthcare workers.

These unique guidelines were not regulatory requirements, as the law enacted under the Clinton Administration had been, but rather performance-based guidelines that the new OSHA chief anticipated would be tried, implemented, and improved upon by those affected. Although these guidelines were directed specifically at nursing homes and long-term care facilities, hospitals were also expected to follow them, as demonstrated by the inclusion of hospitals on the list of places targeted by OSHA for inspection for ergonomics violations. The selection of targeted facilities was based on an injury and illness–reporting rate higher than the national average, which at the time was 8.9 per 100 employees.

OSHA compliance officers were specifically directed to conduct inspections at these noncompliant facilities, with special attention given to reviewing those injuries resulting from ergonomics-related issues. Again, OSHA did not issue citations and penalties based on the ergonomics guidelines, as these were not actionable as specific regulatory requirements. Rather, OSHA inspectors were told to issue the citations and penalties based on the GDC, as was done with the TB requirements, because ergonomics injuries are a recognized hazard in hospitals and nursing homes.

Summary

Overall, the face of the healthcare industry has greatly changed through the incursion of OSHA. The result has been mixed, though certainly one of the positive aspects is highlighting some of the shortcomings of the healthcare industry in providing for the health and safety of its workers.

Further coordination is necessary between the concerns of OSHA inspectors and the practical realities of the hospital environment. In the end, hospitals, once considered an enclave of safety for patients, and by extension, for employees, are now looked upon with more critical eyes by regulators, employees, and patients. OSHA, perhaps like no other agency in history, has changed the appearance of the healthcare landscape as well as the approach that employees and the public take toward healthcare organizations.

Chapter

2

Setting up
a safety program:
How OSHA fits in

Setting up a safety program: How OSHA fits in

Setting up a safety program requires a lot of work, including concentration, attention to detail, and cooperation from both management and employees. Perhaps most of all, it requires an understanding of what it means to ensure that the healthcare environment that you work in is free from recognized hazards.

OSHA's requirements are a good starting point for developing your safety program, but probably will not provide the complete answer to your worker safety needs. Many safety programs will need to take steps beyond what OSHA requires. Do not be afraid to do so with your program. In addition, although OSHA designates many requirements regarding healthcare, its inspectors may cite and fine you for any safety transgressions that may be evident under the proviso of its general duty clause (GDC). Examples of areas in which OSHA could fine you, even though specific regulations do not exist, include the management and risks associated with tuberculosis (TB), ergonomics, and indoor air quality. It is important to recognize that OSHA's regulations are limited, and that your education and training program needs to include a wide range of topics, even beyond the scope of OSHA's specific regulations.

Getting started

In order to start developing your safety program, you need to understand the hazards that could occur in your healthcare environment. You must also understand the nature of these hazards, the potential consequences of exposure to them, and the risks of providing inadequate protection and education for the workforce about hazards in your facility. One way to acquire such information is to read the literature and reports published by federal agencies, such as the National Institute for Occupational Safety and Health, or those published by the American Society of Safety Engineers, the American Industrial Hygiene Association, or the American Conference of Governmental Industrial Hygienists. Also consider reading the *Journal of Occupational and Environmental Medicine*, published by the American College of Occupational and Environmental Medicine, and the *Journal of Toxicology*, published by Dekker.

Within the framework of your organization, you should make it a practice to review your facility's previous injury and illness reports and speak with employees to gain their insights as to both how and under what circumstances injuries are likely to occur, and how to prevent such injuries from occurring in the future, based on their experiences. Most healthcare organizations collect a great deal of quality and incident/variance reporting data. Try to make use of these information resources—there is generally some historical/hazard information to be gleaned from their review. Along with these reviews and interviews, conduct a survey of your facility by performing a walk-through and observing the tasks that employees perform on a daily basis.

Gathering this information will, among other things, provide you with an overview of the hazards that employees routinely encounter. This data collection will also allow you to determine which tasks are the most hazardous and which are the least. Observing employees at work will also help you to determine what factors may make a task more or less hazardous, and whether you could make changes to reduce the hazardous nature of some of the tasks.

Even if some of this information exists at your facility from previous investigations, you will still need to discover for yourself the hazards employees face in your facility. Some of the hazards you will encounter might be considered universal in all health-care environments, such as ergonomic hazards or needlestick injury hazards. Some healthcare environments may have their own specific hazards. For example, facilities that specialize in cancer treatment might be concerned about employee exposure to radioactive materials from therapeutic injections of the isotopes used to treat cancer. Regardless of the nature of these hazards, it is of critical importance for you, as the safety professional, to be fully versed in the presence—actual or potential—of hazardous conditions and practices in your organization.

Understanding the hazards

There are only a few ways that you will come to recognize, identify, and understand which hazards your environment could contain. One way is through experience on the job and the wisdom gleaned from past problems. Some learning will occur through trial and error, no matter how hard you try to prevent problems. The other way to learn about the hazards in your facility, which will help to shorten the experiential pathway, is to preemptively conduct a survey by observing employee actions such as lifting or moving patients or giving injections. In addition, check whether employees who handle hazardous chemicals appropriately make use of material safety data sheets during their regular work activities (see Figure 2.1 "Inspection Checklist" at the end of this chapter).

As a next step, you will need to learn the hazard's potential for harm and how to prioritize strategies for managing those hazards. There are a number of ways to learn about the potential harm that a hazard may pose, from reading a scientific article to reviewing your organization's injury and illness records. Based on the information you have collected, develop a grid that compares the frequency with which hazardous chemicals are used or hazardous tasks are performed with the level of injury that could occur. You can assign ranking based on the level and frequency of risk, and use the ranking to designate your priorities. This list of priorities could then shape program areas such as training, budget requests, and the need for personal protective equipment.

In some cases, you may need to educate employees to defuse their perceptions of the harm that may come from an activity in the facility. For example, when asbestos removal occurs in one area of your facility, does the removal pose a true hazard? Are there safety precautions in place that employees should know about? How do you educate employees about these safety precautions and their effectiveness in reducing or eliminating harm resulting from the removal of the asbestos? Who in your facility should be involved in the removal process? If you do not understand the nuances of asbestos removal, the requirements surrounding its removal, and the way the hazards of asbestos removal are minimized through local and state regulations, in concert with OSHA requirements, then you may have difficulty providing an appropriate response to staff concerns. A wealth of knowledge is available regarding any number of safety topics, both on the Internet and in the person of qualified contractors, asbestos abatement being just an example. Any time you can identify a learning opportunity, act on that opportunity—it will increase your value to yourself and to the organization as a safety professional.

How to monitor your safety program

The next step in setting up a program is to use the data that you have collected. Apply this data in conjunction with a practice that is recognized as appropriate to protect workers and allows them to perform their work effectively and without significant disruption or interference. Do not consider your program as a stagnant document. Regulations change, perceptions change, and most importantly the implementation of the program will change as you gain more experience with it and identify improvement opportunities.

OSHA and the Joint Commission on Accreditation of Healthcare Organizations (JCAHO) share a common concern for the safety of employees. These two agencies also have a requirement to monitor the effects and implementation of your programming so that you can collect data and learn from and improve what you are doing. Failure to monitor your program could lead to JCAHO sanctions, such as Type I violations, and perhaps a loss of accreditation, which then affects insurance reimbursements, such as Medicare and Medicaid, and the stature of the organization in the community. Failure to monitor and evaluate your safety program as a function of OSHA compliance can also have significant results, such as increased inspections, citations, and fines, in addition to loss of respect for the healthcare organization by both your own employees and the community.

The true reason for monitoring, however, should never be to fend off OSHA or the JCAHO. Conduct monitoring to ensure that you properly manage your safety programs and that you appropriately protect employees from workplace hazards and unhealthful exposures.

JCAHO surveyors are more than familiar with the primary OSHA standards we have been discussing and will note violations of those standards as they are encountered during the survey process. The nature of the JCAHO's function is to ensure that each accredited healthcare organization provides safe, appropriate care to patients. An important aspect of that charge is ensuring that each organization provides an appropriate environment for the delivery of care, including safety of all concerned. While JCAHO does provide oversight as a patient-focused function, OSHA, on the other hand, does not get involved with the patient perspective at all, or for the safety of visitors or guests to your facility. OSHA's sole focus is worker health and safety. This is an important distinction that is often overlooked or not understood by hospital employees, visitors, or guests.

It is important to develop effective, well-planned programs to monitor the effects of your safety program. Monitoring ensures that employees are not exposed to hazardous levels of chemicals and that your program is making effective inroads in the workplace. It verifies that employees are becoming more compliant over time with the elements of your program (see Figure 2.2 "Compliance Checklist" at the end of this chapter to assist you in assessing the level of compliance).

Employee performance

A key element in any hospital safety program is, for example, fire safety. Everyone in healthcare recognizes the importance of this program and usually is sensitive to its needs. But how many employees realize that several components of the fire safety program, including training, the use of fire extinguishers, and the establishment of fire brigades, exist as components of various OSHA standards? For personnel to be ready in the event of a fire, they must be educated and trained in the different types of fire extinguishers that are available in the facility, the types of fires such extinguishers effectively combat, and how to use those extinguishers if the need arises. These are OSHA requirements that often get lumped into JCAHO requirements. It is not only good practice to train employees in all of these elements, but also to monitor the way employees use extinguishers and their knowledge of extinguishers' use and purpose.

There are a variety of techniques for monitoring employee performance in fire safety. One method is to observe employees, as required by the JCAHO, as they respond to a mock fire drill. Do the employees know what the protocol is for responding to a drill? Select a mock scenario that would require employees to choose an appropriate extinguisher to put out a fire. In training sessions, conduct demonstrations on the proper use of a fire extinguisher. Make extinguishers available to employees so they can get a feel for how the extinguishers actually work. Employees are often unsure about how to use an extinguisher, or even where to begin. Observation and training provides them with a valuable lesson.

Keep records of the training and monitoring of these programs. Maintain written education plans that outline your teaching topics and identify the important points of the lesson. Keep the education plans on file along with the names of employees you trained (see Figure 2.3 at the end of this chapter for a sample safety education plan). When the inspector arrives at your facility, your documentation will show the steps you took to educate and monitor your employees' activities. Such a proactive approach will often help reduce the number of times inspectors come onto your premises and perform inspections. This approach should also help reduce the number of citations and fines OSHA issues your facility.

Hazard Communication standard

One overlooked area of OSHA training and monitoring is the Hazard Communication standard. Some safety personnel do not think that employees such as clerks, secretaries, and messengers need training in this standard, its applications, and its requirements. Certainly, employees who use chemicals on a routine basis would receive training different from that provided to secretaries and clerks. Yet OSHA inspectors will almost always ask to see evidence of your hazard communication program, the training records that accompany it, and your material safety data sheets (MSDS). The expectation is that each member of the organization will have appropriate training. Because hazard communication is primarily a performance standard, it becomes your responsibility to determine what appropriate training represents for everyone in your facility. Everyone in the organization will require some level of training, even if they are not directly involved with your organization's most hazardous materials. If a material has an MSDS, then there is a training requirement for staff who come into contact with it.

Failure to maintain a hazard communication program and monitor adherence to it at all levels has made this standard the third most often cited standard in healthcare, with fines totaling over $1.3 million in 2003, according to OSHA statistics.

Providing employees with a written document explaining your facility's safety program will be an ineffective measure unless you take additional action to ensure employees understand the safety program and how it affects them on the job. Any time you interface with staff—during fire and other emergency drills, safety rounds, etc.—represents an opportunity to assess their safety competencies and provide excellent data for evaluating your program. Interaction with staff on an ongoing basis should be considered a fundamental component of your safety program.

You should conduct monitoring in a number of ways as well. Firsthand observation is one way of monitoring. However, health and safety professionals in most situations typically have limited time to do this on their own. This is especially true if you have a small facility with little staff, or as is often the case, no support or ancillary staff. Observation and monitoring of program effectiveness and compliance falls upon the shoulders of others in the organization, such as members of the safety committee, department heads, and managers. In some instances you may be able to develop a cadre of trained personnel who act as area or unit safety officers, and who you train to oversee certain activities, including observation and data collection. All of these people must report back to the safety director so that he or she has a perspective of where the programs are succeeding and where they need help. Remember, the goal of the monitoring effort is not to create a "safety police" presence so much as it is to create a team of cooperative individuals who can help you be more effective and efficient in your role.

You could also conduct after-the-fact monitoring by reviewing the injury and illness report logs, and performing investigations of major or significant events immediately after they occur. Such events could include fires, chemical spills in patient areas, or injuries to workers that involve hospitalization or significant lost time on the job. Although not a proactive activity, after-the-fact monitoring does help you to get a better picture of what is happening in your facility, and perhaps gives you a better understanding of what went wrong so that you can address the situation and correct it.

Some safety professionals also try to include "near misses" in their overview of the safety programs to address accidents that were averted in some manner. Developing a system of reporting near misses can be an invaluable proactive measure in accident prevention.

Ensuring compliance

It is unlikely that you will ever ensure compliance absolutely. People mean well, and they usually try to do the right thing. Employees do not want to be injured on the job, nor do they wish to be exposed to hazardous chemicals or infectious agents. You cannot ensure that employees are always wearing their respirators appropriately and under the right circumstances, and you cannot be certain that employees are always wearing protective gloves, lab coats, and eyewear, because you cannot be everywhere at once. However, you can take steps to further minimize the possibility of employee noncompliance.

Ensuring compliance requires that you enlist and receive the aid of employees and supervisors throughout the facility. Although punitive measures are often counterproductive in achieving compliance, there are ways to help add an extra measure of support to ensure employee compliance. One way to accomplish this is through the use of your organization's employee evaluation process. Enlist your institution to add a section on safety compliance to the employee review form.

Raises and promotions are typically a function of the performance of an employee in his or her job. You do not want to punish an employee for getting injured or being exposed to a chemical on the job. However, you can use the review process (remember this is another instance in which there is a direct interaction with an employee) to ensure that employees actively and routinely participate in safety training and education. Let employees know that their compliance with the safety program plays a role in their overall job performance, thus qualifying them for raises, bonuses, and promotions, in a similar fashion to the way attendance, punctuality, and job performance do. This approach can help you increase the chances of safety compliance significantly.

Employees often see safety measures as tasks that will weigh them down. Discourage this type of negative attitude and work to develop an attitude of enlightenment and participation. One school of thought states that safety on the job is in large measure due to behavioral changes in employees. Not everyone is a behaviorist, but each of us can assist employees in learning the safe way to do a job. We should be able to help employees realize that doing the job safely is easy, and that the benefits of working safely far exceed those of not doing so.

Liability under OSHA

Construction

This category includes both new construction and renovation projects. In either case, the healthcare organization may hire an outside contractor to perform the work, including demolition, asbestos removal, and refitting of the new or renovated facility. What happens if there is a workplace accident or a violation of some other OSHA standard involving the contractor's employees? Who is responsible?

If the contractor is responsible for the construction or renovation site and has his or her own employees and subcontractors on the job, working with the OSHA inspector and handling the complaint and any subsequent actions or fines will typically be the responsibility of the contractor. However, the OSHA inspector has the authority to include the hospital in its citation, if he or she believes the hospital chose a contractor who was not adequately prepared to perform the work or was not capable of doing the work in such a manner as to appropriately protect hospital employees. An example of this type of situation might involve contractors who are not certified by state or local agencies, and therefore, generally are not qualified to do the work. Often, the results will be fines all around.

Bloodborne pathogens and needlestick prevention

The Bloodborne Pathogen (BBP) standard has been in existence since 1991. However, after 10 years, evidence indicated that needlesticks and contaminated sharps were the major sources of employee exposure to BBPs. In 2001, OSHA revised and updated the standard to reflect these findings.

The revised BBP standard added new terms that clarified the definition of sharps with engineered sharps injury protection and needleless systems. In addition, there were new sections of the law requiring an exposure control plan in which employers must take into account any changes in technology that could lead to the reduction or elimination of employee exposure to BBPs. The revised regulation made clear in the requirement that "frontline" employees be active participants in the selection process for new needlestick prevention devices. And, finally, the revision required healthcare organizations to include documentation of the process by which devices were selected or eliminated for consideration for use in the hospital.

These latter elements, along with the existing requirements of the Bloodborne Pathogen standard, have made the enforcement of this standard and a review of its requirements a key component of OSHA inspection activities. In fact, this standard represented the number one cited standard in hospitals in 2003, according to OSHA statistics.

Engineering controls

The identification and implementation of engineering controls is the first step toward eliminating or minimizing your employees' risks of exposure to BBPs. The Bloodborne Pathogen standard (29 CFR 1910.1030) defines engineering controls as "controls (e.g., sharps disposal containers, self-sheathing needles, safer medical devices, such as sharps with engineered sharps injury protections and needleless systems) that isolate or remove the bloodborne pathogens hazard from the workplace." This is the foundation upon which the success of your exposure control activities depends.

Work practice controls

Work practice controls or administrative actions are defined in the standard as "controls that reduce the likelihood of exposure by altering the manner in which a task is performed (e.g., prohibiting recapping of needles by a two-handed technique)." These controls provide for the determination of "hazardous" activities that cannot otherwise be mitigated through engineering controls and the obligation to provide guidelines or oversight for the utilization of reduced-risk practices.

Personal protective equipment

The use of personal protective equipment (PPE) is a serious step in employee protection. On the hierarchy of protective measures, it is the last resort. Some tasks require the use of PPE in combination with engineering controls or administrative action, such as mandating the use of respirators by staff members who are exposed to patients with active TB. Yet the use of PPE has become a key method of exposure protection for employees in healthcare facilities everywhere.

Using OSHA's PPE requirements, conduct an assessment to determine the hazard, the level of exposure, and the appropriate pieces of protective equipment. Using PPE comes with responsibilities and requirements, including the need to educate and train your employees in their use of such equipment and ensuring that it works and fits correctly.

In some cases, OSHA requires medical testing and evaluation of employees both prior to their using PPE and on a regular basis (usually annually) thereafter. Such testing could include taking an employee's medical history, including any history of smoking or allergies. The examination could also include a pulmonary function test to determine how well the employee's lungs are working and whether he or she could tolerate using a respirator. Conducting hearing testing and establishing baseline auditory levels are important in determining the hearing capacity of employees who use loud equipment, and in doing so could also help track the effectiveness of the hearing protection equipment.

Respirators

The practice of providing healthcare workers with devices, specifically respirators, to protect them from exposure to hazards such as TB is relatively new. Certainly, we are all familiar with the use of surgical masks to protect patients from employees. Now, for perhaps the first time in our history, we are protecting employees from patients.

Healthcare workers should be familiar with the terms "fit testing," "negative pressure and positive pressure respirators," and "high efficiency particulate air" filters, along with N95 respirators. The concern about respirators stems from a Centers for Disease Control and Prevention (CDC) advisory issued in 1994 about how to protect workers from exposure to TB. OSHA attempted to step in on this guideline and create a regulation to make such protective measures mandatory. OSHA's six-year effort to enact this legislation failed. However, in order to ensure that healthcare institutions adhere to the CDC guidelines, OSHA has elected to continue to enforce the CDC guidelines for TB protection and to use the GDC to cite and fine employers who do not conform.

Healthcare employees who provide care to TB patients are not the only healthcare workers who must use respirators. Some healthcare providers who work with other hazardous agents, such as the drugs that treat respiratory syncytial virus, must use respirators when handling these drugs.

Some maintenance workers also must wear respirators. These workers need protection against such materials as chemicals, asbestos, or hazardous fumes from acid neutralization tanks. Maintenance workers who wear respirators are usually covered by specific OSHA standards. These standards could include the asbestos standard, or the standards for protection against specific chemicals, such as acids, corrosives, or even radioactive materials, if part of an employee's job requires going onto the roof near fume hood exhausts that emit radionuclides.

In each case, the requirements for respirator use call for the development of a respirator program. This program should include the requirements for selecting a respirator based on an analysis of the hazards. In some cases, measurement of the potential levels of exposure to the hazard will also be necessary. The program should include the necessary requirements for medical clearance, fit testing, and education and training.

Prior to the time when OSHA rescinded its proposed TB standard, a separate section covered TB respirators and other types of respirators. Currently, however, all respirator requirements fall under one standard, 29 CFR 1910.134. Hospitals often find this standard problematic, particularly the portion concerning medical clearance and fit testing of TB respirators, because most healthcare institutions do not understand the nature of the respirator requirements, the meaning of fit testing, and how it applies to them and their employees. In addition, the number of employees who must be medically cleared and fit tested, especially in the larger teaching hospitals in urban centers, plus the amount of both ongoing and renewed training, creates a large obstacle in terms of facility resources.

Note that if your maintenance staff wear respirators when working near asbestos or fume hood exhaust stacks, the requirements for fit testing and medical clearance of those employees are often more stringent than the TB requirements.

Gloves, goggles, and other protective eyewear

The use of gloves for personal protection has become a significant issue in healthcare over the past several years. Glove selection, including for protection against exposure to BBPs, has become a sophisticated and complex task. Many safety and healthcare professionals have seen changes in both types and availability of gloves over time. One such change came as a result of healthcare workers experiencing serious, even career-ending, allergic reactions to latex gloves. Yet latex is one of the key materials that provide protection against BBPs. Alternate gloves are also available now for use by employees in protecting themselves against exposures to BBPs, including "low-latex" gloves that are powder-free. Often healthcare providers on the clinical units will use vinyl gloves when their duties do not involve potential exposure to BBPs.

Other types of gloves are in use throughout the hospital environment. Those who deal with caustic chemicals and cleaning agents often use thick rubber gloves. Workers who use cryogenic materials or those who must deal with sterilizers will use special protective gloves made of thick cotton or other materials to prevent either freeze burns or steam burns.

Although OSHA has no *specific* standard for glove use, it requires an employer to provide appropriate PPE when necessary to its employees. OSHA does not define the exact circumstances under which employees should use gloves. It leaves that determination up to the discretion of the user. Establish a glove-use policy to avoid any confusion within your facility. OSHA also provides nonmandatory standards for selecting the proper PPE. Once again, OSHA could cite a facility under the GDC for failure to follow its general glove-use requirements.

Additional safeguards

Fume hoods and biosafety cabinets

In order to protect employees from exposure to hazardous chemicals or biological agents, in many cases you must provide certain engineering controls to ensure an appropriate environment for conducting these types of activities. In instances in which chemical fume hoods are indicated, you must make sure that the hoods provide the appropriate level of airflow (*note:* See *Industrial Ventilation: A Manual of Recommended Practices,* 25th edition, 2004, American Conference of Governmental Industrial Hygienists, Cincinnati). In situations that require biosafety cabinets, the cabinets must work correctly as specified in the manufacturer's manual (see also *Primary Containment of Biohazards: Selection, Installation and Use of Biological Safety Cabinets,* CDC/NIH Publication, September 1995). Remember that these types of equipment are not to be used interchangeably. Biosafety cabinets are not designed to protect workers from exposure to hazardous chemicals; using them for this purpose can result in a hazard significantly greater than the hazard you are trying to control.

Biosafety cabinets are designed to ensure that microbial agents used in research are not exposed to the environment in general, thus protecting them from becoming infected. More importantly, however, biosafety cabinets ensure that workers are not exposed to the agents being used in the enclosures, such as microbes, infectious agents, or chemotherapeutic drugs.

The OSHA Laboratory standard (29CFR1910.1450) provides performance-based requirements for laboratories to follow to ensure that proper policies and procedures are developed and put in place to protect workers from exposure to hazardous materials, whether they are chemical, biological, or pharmaceutical in nature.

It is left up to each institution to develop programs that demonstrate compliance with the regulatory requirements of this standard, including the appointment of a chemical hygiene officer who is responsible for program implementation, either in each laboratory or in laboratories throughout the facility.

Although the Laboratory Standard is performance based, it includes a number of topics that need to be covered in each laboratory plan, including hazard communication, fume hood maintenance, and exposure prevention.

TB protection

TB remains a significant focus of OSHA, even though most of the components of that program are primarily derived from the CDC's guidelines. Even so, there are elements, such as respiratory protection, that fall within OSHA's direct purview. You can almost be assured, particularly if you are located in a community with a high prevalence of TB, that OSHA will look at your TB exposure control plan as part of any inspection.

Ergonomics

As discussed in Chapter one, there is no OSHA ergonomics standard. Recognizing the prevalence of ergonomic injuries in healthcare, it is incumbent on healthcare organizations to develop strategies for appropriately managing employee safety as a function of ergonomic concerns. The most compelling reasons for doing this are, of course, the importance of maintaining a healthy and productive workforce. Musculoskeletal disorders (e.g., ergonomic injuries in the workplace) represent a significant potential for reduced productivity as well as increased operating costs related to higher insurance and workers' compensation premiums. Tie these elements in with an aging employee population and the relevance of ergonomic awareness is readily seen.

OSHA will hold you accountable for how your organization manages (reduction/prevention) musculoskeletal disorders. In fact, if you look at your injury and illness logs for OSHA recordable cases, you will see a separate column for just this type of injury. In the past, OSHA has used this data to target various healthcare facilities for inspections and there is every indication that this practice will continue. If an inspection took place and you could not demonstrate your success in correcting the deficits, or failed to show a good-faith effort to correct them, OSHA might very well cite you under the GDC.

Training

Education and training are key components of virtually every OSHA-mandated program, including hazard communication, respiratory protection, and BBPs. It is important that you understand the key training elements for each OSHA-required program and how to develop programming that will keep you compliant.

Create a lesson plan for each training program that includes subjects to be covered, learning objectives, and even pre- and post-tests to help you evaluate initial and ongoing competency. Keep the lesson plan on file to use as a demonstration of compliance with training requirements for each of the OSHA programs in the event of an inspection.

Lesson plans are not sufficient in and of themselves to maintain compliance with education requirements. To complete the compliance equation, you must execute your training plan and document the name and identification number of each participant. Inspectors have been known to back-check this kind of information, as well as to question employees whom you indicated attended the program.

As mentioned earlier, consider administering pre- and post-tests as part of your training and education programs. Such tests can be used for fire safety training, as well as for training in hazard communication, chemical safety, or a variety of other areas. The concept comes from educational settings from junior high to college and beyond and is used as the basis for determining the effectiveness of the training and, if employees are involved in repeat training over time, the retention of that knowledge.

Testing also helps establish the credibility of your program. It is a good practice to periodically evaluate the tests themselves. Do they reflect current "core" knowledge expectations? Do they reflect confusion of staff in particular areas? While not exactly a "face-to-face" interaction, any feedback from your "students" can be of great benefit in identifying improvement opportunities for your education programs, and also your safety program in general.

Programming

Establishing programs in each of the areas identified in OSHA's standards is a key step in maintaining compliance. Follow through and document the steps you are taking and why. It is important to note that since many OSHA standards are now performance-based (designed to emphasize the ends and not necessarily the means by which you reach those ends), be sure also to document why you chose to follow one particular method of reaching those ends versus another. This documentation may become important when you have to provide a response to an OSHA complaint, or more importantly, a defense in a post-inspection hearing.

FIGURE
2.1
INSPECTION CHECKLIST

	Y	N	Comments
Programs			
Injury-illness logs			
Summary reports			
Signage			
Exposure monitoring			
Formaldehyde			
Noise			
Asbestos			
Ethylene oxide			
Hazard communication			
Written program			
MSDSs			
Training			
Respiratory protection			
Medical evaluation			
Fit-testing			
Education/training			
Performance evaluation			
Bloodborne pathogens			
Written evaluation/policy			
Labeling			
Sharps containers			
Sharps evaluation program			
Hazardous materials			
Asbestos program			
Ethylene oxide program			
Formaldehyde program			
Glutaraldehyde program			
Chemical waste handling/disposal			
Infectious waste handling/disposal			

	Y	N	Comments
FIGURE 2.1			**INSPECTION CHECKLIST (CONT.)**

	Y	N	Comments
Programs			
Fire safety			
Written plan			
Exit routes			
Fire extinguishers			
Alarm systems			
Sprinkler systems			
Egress doors			
Fire exits			
TB			
Risk analysis			
Written TB program			
Education/training			
Use of PPE			
Ergonomics			
Hazard evaluation			
Lifting policy			
Lifting devices			
Back safety education			
PPE			
Hazard evaluation and analysis			
Selection of PPE			
Respirators			
Goggles/eyewear			
Face shields			
Lab coats			
Gowns			
Gloves			
Heat/cryogenic protection			
Safety shoes			
Laboratory standard			
Written program			
Monitoring			
MSDS's			
PPE			
Hood program			
Warnings			
Education/training			

FIGURE
2.2

COMPLIANCE CHECKLIST

OSHA program

	Program elements	Met Y/N	Suggested corrections
Record-keeping			
	Injury-illness		
	Annual reporting		
Fire prevention			
	Written program		
	Emergency procedures		
	Exit routes marked		
	Fire extinguishers		
	Stand pipes/hoses		
	Alarm systems		
	Code compliance		
	Training/education		
Noise prevention			
	Audiometric testing		
	Hearing protection devices		
	Noise monitoring		
	Education		
"Hazwopper"			
	Training		
	PPE selection		
	Internal disaster response		
	External disaster response		
	WMD response		
PPE			
	PPE selection/approval methods		
	Eye/face protection		
	Skin/mucous membrane protection		
	Head protection		
	Foot protection		
	Gloves (hand protection)		
	Electrical protection		
	Training		
Permit confined spaces			
	Testing methods		
	Written entry procedures		
	Training		
Lock-out/tag-out			
	Written program		
	Identification of spaces		
	Training		
Machine guarding			
	Audit of machines		
	Education/training		
Welding			
	Requirements		
	Permitting		
	Program element training		

FIGURE 2.2	COMPLIANCE CHECKLIST (CONT.)		

OSHA program

	Program elements	Met Y/N	Suggested corrections
Electrical safety			
	Education/training		
Toxic and hazardous materials			
	ID of chemicals in use		
	Specific programs		
	Asbestos		
	Benzene		
	Ethylene oxide		
	Formaldehyde		
	Methylene chloride		
	Monitoring		
	Record-keeping		
	Medical surveillance		
Respiratory protection			
	Respirator selection		
	Medical monitoring		
	Fit testing		
	Education/trailing		
	Observation of workers		
	Written program		
Hazard communication			
	Written program		
	MSDS's		
	Education/training		
Blood borne pathogens			
	Identification of hazards		
	Selection of PPE		
	Needleless device selection		
	Employee participation		
	HBV Immunization program		
	Employee declination process		
	Education/training		
Laboratory standard			
	Written program		
	Monitoring		
	MSDS's		
	PPE		
	Hood program		
	Warnings		
	Education/training		

FIGURE
2.3
SAFETY EDUCATION LESSON PLAN

Safety Education Lesson Plan

Fire safety

Purpose: To teach employees the fire safety plan of _____

After the lesson employees will be able to:

Detail the fire safety plan of _____
- Employees will know the emergency procedures to follow if they discover a fire
- Employees will be familiar with the emergency numbers they must contact
- Employees will know the differences in fire safety procedures on different shifts
- Employees will understand the type of fire hazards at _____
- Employees will be able to explain terms such as protect in place, fire zone, and egress corridor
- Employees will be able to explain what extinguishers are available to them for use
- Employees will be able to describe the method of selection of the appropriate fire extinguisher
- Employees will be able to demonstrate the use of a fire extinguisher

Employee pretest

Describe the fire safety plan for _____

What do you do if you discover a fire?

List three fire hazards you may find at _____

_____   _____   _____

List three differences in emergency fire response on the day shift and the evening shift

_____   _____   _____

What is meant by:
   Fire zone

   Protect in place

   Egress corridor

List two emergency numbers used at _____
_____   _____

Identify the fire extinguishers in use at _____

How do you select which fire extinguisher is appropriate for use in a fire?

Chapter

3

Events that prompt
OSHA action

Events that prompt OSHA action

A variety of events or circumstances could occur that may result in an OSHA visit to your facility. Some of these situations may be beyond your control, but if you establish an effective safety program and prepare diligently for any contingency, you can avoid an OSHA inspection and, as a result, any adverse consequences for you and your facility.

If you undergo an inspection, an important aspect of your preparation is establishing good working relationships with your employees. This may be apparent from your point of view as an employee of the institution. However, the role of safety professionals is sometimes misconstrued and their intentions are not always obvious to the others who work at the facility. It is part of your task as the safety expert to make your goals and intentions clear to employees with whom you work and interact each day so they know you are working in their best interests.

If there is even a slight perception that you are not working your hardest on behalf of the employees to help resolve OSHA-related problems, a concerned employee could contact the local OSHA office to help push you along. If on the other hand, you are perceived as open, honest, and working in the best interests of employees, you will almost certainly get a call before OSHA does. There are never any guarantees, but employees who trust you will usually call you to help with a problem and will not use OSHA as a wedge.

Advance warning?

Generally, OSHA inspectors do not give advance warning of their visits. However, when an employee makes a complaint about a health or safety hazard in the workplace, OSHA inspectors may call your facility's designated officials (e.g., administrator or safety professional) to inform them that a complaint has been made. OSHA will provide a copy of that complaint via the mail or fax. The complaining employee has the right to request that OSHA conduct an inspection, especially if the employee sees the hazard as an imminent threat or danger. The likelihood of your organization receiving a call from OSHA as opposed to an inspection can very much depend on the severity of the condition about which they have received the complaint.

Oftentimes, if the OSHA inspector feels that the condition can be remedied without a site visit, he or she will interact with you remotely. This is not to say that the phone call might not result in an on-site visit if the inspector feels that you have not adequately responded to the complaint.

A similar series of events could also occur in which OSHA receives a complaint about the workplace from someone other than an employee. In other words, if someone enters your facility and observes a condition that he or she feels is unsafe, the person could file a complaint with OSHA. Even more significant is the fact that whether the complaint comes from an employee or another source, the person can make the complaint anonymously. This sometimes works out better for the facility, as OSHA is less likely in the beginning to send out an inspector on an anonymous call.

It is important to remember that OSHA is under no obligation to reveal to you the identity of the complainant, regardless of the complainant's standing—employee, "interested" party, etc.—during the investigation. Though it might not seem so, anonymity is useful for all concerned in that it limits the likelihood of actual or per-ceived acts of reprisal on the part of an employer. As a general rule of thumb, it is rarely a good idea to engage in any activities that could be considered retaliatory. The best tact to take is to identify appropriate improvements or remediations and to monitor for recurrence of noncompliant behavior or conditions.

Other reasons OSHA inspects

If there is a circumstance that requires you to report a problem to OSHA, expect an inspection. These conditions include an employee death on the job or three or more employees injured on the job being admitted to the hospital within 30 days of a single accident.

OSHA inspections could also occur as the result of "programmed" inspections. Such inspections, typically unannounced, occur in industries where there has been a histor-ically high rate of injuries, such as ergonomics injuries in nursing homes, or in indus-tries that are recognized as high-hazard workplaces, including construction sites.

OSHA often designates industries for inspection during a particular calendar year based on a high incidence rate of injuries or illnesses. Recently, OSHA has looked at healthcare facilities, including nursing homes and hospitals, with an injury incidence rate in excess of 8.9 per 100 workers as warranting inspections. The rate was selected as being above the most recently published Bureau of Labor Statistics national average for injuries and illnesses in these workplaces. Of particular relevance to OSHA in selecting healthcare facilities was the increased incidence of ergonomic injuries to employees in these work environments.

Once you have undergone an OSHA inspection, you may be subject to follow-up inspections to ensure that you have taken appropriate steps to prevent similar problems from occurring in the future.

Be aware there are circumstances that could lead to OSHA providing you with advance notice of an inspection, including situations involving union workers. Other circumstances could include situations involving imminent danger that need correcting as quickly as possible, or one involving a fatal accident or catastrophe. Advance notice in these circumstances is necessary to ensure that hospital managers and union representatives, for example, will be present for the inspection.

There also could be circumstances under which an OSHA area director would determine that advanced notice would lead to a more effective inspection. For example, if OSHA is inspecting a report of the staff's failure to wear appropriate personal protective equipment in an operating room that uses ultraviolet lights during certain procedures (e.g., knee or hip replacements), the area director would want the inspector to witness the procedure firsthand because such a procedure is not performed routinely. Advance notice would ensure that the inspector appears at the appropriate time.

What if OSHA is a phone call away?

As indicated previously, many OSHA inspections are conducted without advance warning, or with less than a few hours notice. In many situations, the inspector calls to inform you or hospital administration that a complaint has been filed about a particular problem, such as poor indoor air quality. Likely the call will surprise you because you know absolutely nothing about the problem or the circumstances surrounding the complaint.

Since you have received a phone call, do not squander the opportunity to take a proactive approach to prepare for the inquiry. No matter when the call comes in, investigate the problem firsthand. Do not try to identify who made the complaint. Do not try to assign blame or guilt to anyone. Interview everyone in the affected area, and talk to as many people as you are able from the department and other areas. For example, if there is an air quality complaint, speak to your chief of maintenance or plant engineer to find out about previous air filter or fan problems. They may have even received complaints in the past about the problem and never shared that information with you. Gather as many facts as you can, determine a plan of action, and create a timeline for repairing the problem.

Next, respond to the inspector in writing and by phone as soon as possible. Typically, you will be given only a few days to respond, but you will be able to propose a timeline for repairing or resolving the problem, as long as it is reasonable and gets to the heart of the matter in an effective fashion. Do not present lack of money as an excuse for not fixing the problem; OSHA is concerned with the safety of your facility, not its financial state.

How to respond when an OSHA inspector arrives

When the OSHA inspector arrives at your facility, do not panic. There are a number of crucial steps to follow. First, do not leave the inspector alone to tour the facility unaccompanied. Also, even though the law allows you to ask the inspector to leave and provide a warrant to enter and search the premises, the best advice is to accommodate the inspector. The inspector will likely get the warrant almost immediately, and will be back on your doorstep later that day, or the next day for certain. You will have accomplished nothing, as the problem that the inspector is there to review will not, in all likelihood, have been remedied. In most cases, the end result of refusing entry to the inspector is a much less friendly and uncooperative inspector ready to do the same job.

The inspector will identify him or herself, and will show you his or her credentials. As you take the inspector to the administrator's office, make sure that you have already done your homework. By this I mean have a phone tree set up, starting with your secretary or hospital administrator to inform all department heads that there is an OSHA inspector on the premises. It probably will not lead to a mitigation of the problem that the inspector came to look at, but it might prevent the inspector from finding other problems. For example, is your oxygen cylinder storage system compliant? Are they chained and stored properly or are there cylinders lying around on the floor?

Problems like this occur every day, but can be rapidly fixed. You have then taken a little of the edge off of not having received advanced notice. Even though you have a problem, you were able to address it before it affects the current inspection.

As you take the inspector through the hospital to the administrator's office, or after the initial meeting, to the location of the complaint, try to be as thoughtful as you can about the route you take. Try to go through areas that you know are secure, that is, where the managers and department heads run a tight operation and keep their units in excellent condition and in compliance with the regulations—as you have educated them. OSHA inspectors are obligated to cite any problems that they find, even though they are in the facility for another purpose. A simple inspection for one problem can escalate into a major event.

It is important to remember that if inspectors do identify unsafe or unhealthy work conditions during the walk-through, they may offer technical advice on how to eliminate hazards. One word of caution—this is not the time to argue with the inspector. Anything you can do to correct discrepancies on the spot will work toward demonstration of "good faith" determinations when the inspector (and others) is making an assessment of findings and penalties.

The following is an example of a situation in which an OSHA inspector was on-site investigating the shooting death of an employee at a facility, and while there, observed other OSHA violations:

> Even though the inspector was focused on the workplace violence that resulted in the death of one worker, on his way to the site of the shooting, he observed a worker from the facility's electrical shop stringing wire through the ceiling. Interested,

he stopped to take a look at what was going on and observed asbestos above the ceiling exactly in the spot where the employee was pulling the wire. He then asked the worker whether he had received training in asbestos-related work, whether he had been provided with a respirator, and whether he had received training and procedures on setting up a safe work area. The answers were almost immaterial, as he had already observed the employee doing this work without any personal protective equipment, such as a respirator, and without any protective barriers to shield other employees from exposure to asbestos that could become loose during the course of the job. The OSHA compliance officer wrote his first citation at that moment, moved on to investigating the shooting, and came back a week later to delve further into the facility's asbestos policies and procedures and employee training.

In the end, you need to be honest with inspectors when they question you. However, you do not need to volunteer information unnecessarily. Do not respond to a question that you have not been asked.

What the inspector looks for

Generally, inspectors will look at the problem that they were sent to investigate. However, the inspector will also routinely look at some other program items. First, the inspector will want to review your injury and illness reporting log. In addition, the inspector will want to make sure that the appropriate reporting documents, including the annual report of injuries and illnesses, are posted in a location accessible to employees. Remember, in a large facility you may need to post this documentation in a number of places to ensure that all employees see it. The inspector will also want to ensure that OSHA form No. 3165, which explains an employee's safety and health rights, is posted in a location visible to all employees.

The inspector will follow this by reviewing your written hazard communication program. Inspectors are directed to routinely look at that program whenever they conduct an inspection. The program, you will recall, must include a list of all hazardous chemicals in the workplace by location, and describe the way in which you intend to transmit information about the hazards of those chemicals to your employees. Again, in a large institution, you may need to specifically list hazardous chemicals by the exact location in which they will be found.

If inspectors find a problem or are unconvinced you are fulfilling the requirements of the law, they may broaden the inspection and include issues other than those that first brought them to the facility. For example, if the injury and illness log appears to be underreported or if there seems to be an excess of cases (especially involving musculoskeletal injuries), the inspector could decide to dig deeper into the matter. The inspector could question employees of different units, including speaking with union representatives, who are required by law to be included in the proceedings.

Similarly, if your hazard communication program is deficient in some way, such as a failure to list all of the hazardous chemicals in the facility, or if the training program appears inadequate, OSHA could launch a broader investigation into your training and education for OSHA programs generally. In the process, the inspector could uncover additional programmatic problems that OSHA will need to investigate.

The inspector may come into the facility to investigate one complaint, but a failure on your part to have your programming and other materials in good shape, readily accessible, and easily understood, can lead to a larger investigation—and a bigger problem for you and your facility.

How staff figure into an inspection

The staff in your facility can be your friends or your worst nightmare. Some employees are content to work within the system and use the safety professional or whatever other means are offered to help identify and resolve problems. Other staff members will want nothing to do with the system in place, and will purposely look to cause problems. This means that if a safety or health issue bothers them, this latter group will never turn to you for assistance or report a problem to you. Their primary means of getting a problem out in the open will be to call a regulatory agency, most often OSHA. Such people are rarely happy or satisfied with the outcome. Often, these individuals have other problems with their supervisor, administrator, or even a fellow employee, and they are using the immediate concern as a way of venting and expressing other frustrations. Sometimes, these individuals do not even realize what they are doing or why they are doing it.

All of this points to the fact that, as stated previously, you need to not only perform your job with excellence, but also develop a corps of cooperative employees who can help you better understand the problems in their area, and who can help you resolve these problems. You should not expect, nor develop, this corps of individuals to be "snitches." Rather, you should develop them to be assistants in understanding the concerns and needs of the employees with respect to health and safety in each area of the facility and to act as advocates for the safety of all.

Finally, you must realize that the OSHA inspector can, and most likely will, interview employees during the course of the inspection. As a safety professional or administrator, you will not be allowed into the interview room. Everything that is said is private and confidential, but goes a long way in helping inspectors make some decisions about how their findings add up in the face of the information they obtain during the interviews.

Ultimately, your staff can be very instrumental in determining the outcome of any OSHA inspection.

Union workers and OSHA

Many healthcare institutions in the United States have union employees working in them, including nurses, housekeepers, materials handlers, security officers, and others. Unions represent their employees and work on their behalf in a number of arenas—health and safety being among the more important. There are many opinions and prejudices that exist among administrators, safety professionals, and other nonunion hospital employees who must work with those who are represented by unions. Sometimes the relationships among these groups are contentious at best and oftentimes, during a problem these relationships can become strained. As a safety professional, you must consider your position in the organization.

Make it clear that your role is to ensure that everyone knows about the facility's safety program and its policies, and that if a question arises, you will make decisions and judgments based on the facts, no matter what those facts may be, and whether they come out on the employee's side or the employer's side. This position may sound simplistic, but it often becomes a complex and contentious issue as the union personnel may see your efforts as anti-worker, and nonunion workers or administrators may see your efforts as capitulating to the union position on whatever the issue is at hand. For example, working to establish a no-lift policy could be construed by unions as trying to eliminate some jobs, while administrators could see it as an attempt to soothe union pressures. Your goal is to establish yourself as a neutral party whose interests are safety and nothing more.

As time goes on, the wisdom of this position becomes more and more evident, especially if there are complaints that bring in OSHA and involve employee interviews and union involvement in the walk-through of the facility and in the interviews. The employees are going to be more honest and less judgmental if they understand that you are a fair and true representative of safety, regardless of where the chips may fall in terms of the findings of the inspection.

Appropriate actions during an OSHA visit

When inspectors arrive at your facility, they should present you with their credentials and provide you with a reason for the visit. Hold an initial meeting that includes the safety professional, a senior administrator, and the head of the department from which the complaint stems. If the complaint involved air quality, you might want to include the head of maintenance, or if it originated in a patient care area, invite a representative of nursing. In addition, make sure that a union representative is present if you have a union on-site.

As pointed out previously, OSHA inspectors may question employees. Although employees could have their union representative in the room during questioning, neither you nor any member of administration can be present. This is often a difficult role to accept, but remember you cannot discuss any aspects of the interview with the employee, either before or after the fact. You may, however, get a chance later to rebut information provided if it becomes an important matter in the final adjudication of the inspection.

Always tell the inspector the truth, but do not volunteer information, and do not answer more than you were specifically asked. If the inspector asks a question, make your answer succinct and to the point. If you are uncertain about the meaning or purpose of the question, ask the inspector to clarify before you attempt to answer.

When inspectors are in your facility, they will typically bring a camera and take photos of certain items pertaining to the investigation. Make sure you take the same photos with your camera. Also, be sure to take notes. Write down any comments or observations that the inspector makes. Inspectors will review with you the bulk of their findings, although not citations or penalties, at the end of the day. Do not rely on a closing conference to provide you with all the information from the day's inspection. By taking your own notes, you will be in a much better position to evaluate OSHA's findings in relation to your perception of events.

Handling extended OSHA inspections

Inspections can last for one, two, or even several days, or sometimes even up to a month or more. The thought of this type of an inspection lasting for an extended period of time is daunting, to be sure. But do not be defeated or manipulated by a lengthy inspection. Make sure that you have a meeting place each day where you can greet the inspector and accompany him or her to an office for an opening conference. Make sure that you and the inspector agree upon an agenda for each day. It would be best if you could get the inspector to agree upon an agenda for the next day during the previous evening's closing conference. This will allow you to give advanced notice to department heads in the areas where the inspector will be visiting the next day.

And even though after a period of time inspectors will become more familiar to you and a bit less intimidating, remember that just like you, they have a job to do. Inspectors will not forget that job just because you have gotten to know each other a little better.

It is true that you have additional responsibilities in your job beyond working with the OSHA inspector. However, it is in your best interest to be with the inspector as much as possible, and to delegate other responsibilities to your staff, if possible. If not, speak with your senior administrator to find others who can handle any tasks that cannot be delayed. If there are matters that you need to deal with during the inspector's visit, do so after inspection hours, if possible, or during scheduled breaks. Never take a phone call and discuss any private hospital business in the presence of the inspector. Do not give the inspector a reason to acquire additional information that could be harmful to your cause.

Can you prevent a citation from being issued?

Whether you can prevent a citation from being issued is largely dependent on the inspector. If you can resolve the problem or any other violation that came to the attention of the inspector during the visit while he or she is still on-site, the chances of avoiding the citation or having a citation issued without an accompanying penalty increases.

During the closing conference, the inspector will outline the unsafe or unhealthy conditions identified during the inspection and explain which violations may be cited. At this time, you will have the opportunity to provide any documentation that demonstrates your compliance efforts or that may assist OSHA in making a determination of the time needed for abatement of the hazards. It is important to note that every organization has the right to appeal OSHA citations. The appeal process may have any number of results from reduction of fines to removal of violations. It is a crucial component of this process that you make a considered evaluation of the appeal process and determine its efficacy for your organization.

If you have a violation that is not easily corrected, ensure that you resolve it in as timely a fashion as possible. While you may get some indication from the inspector as to a likely hazard abatement schedule, it is always better to correct deficiencies sooner rather than later. Early resolution is a powerful demonstrator of the effectiveness of your safety program and the extent to which safety pervades the organization.

That notwithstanding, the resolution will often involve money and time, and perhaps even education of the staff on such matters as how to label chemicals in accordance with the Hazard Communication standard or how to set up a protective barrier during asbestos-related projects. If that is the case, be sure to give yourself enough time to deal with these issues and to actually resolve the problem, because in all likelihood, the inspector will come back. If the inspector does not see progress or a good faith effort, then the violation will likely become more severe and result in increased penalties and fines.

Receipt of a citation

Receipt of a citation could vary from a few days to even weeks. The problem is not really the details of the citation, as oftentimes the inspector will give you an inkling of what violations to expect at the closing conference, or even during the walk-through itself.

The delay in receiving the citation is usually the result of OSHA deciding on penalties. The decisions about penalties, and even the citations, reside with OSHA senior level personnel, usually the area administrator, and not with the inspector. However, the inspector certainly has input into these decisions. Part of that input is based on the experience the inspector has on the site visit.

If your facility receives a citation and penalty, OSHA delivers it to you by certified letter. At the same time, the OSHA regional office will send a press release to local media about the action, the penalty, and the fine. Typically, administration or public relations officials handle press releases. However, if a call should make it through to your office, be polite, but do not respond to any questions unless specifically authorized to do so by your administration. The best advice for handling these callers is to refer them to the public relations office, if you have one, or to administration. At the same time, you should educate administration and the public relations office about OSHA's findings.

Chapter
4

Responding to citations and penalties

Responding to citations and penalties

Act immediately

As discussed in Chapter 3, the citation, along with the penalty, will arrive by certified mail within a few days to a few weeks after the inspection ends. The citation will specify the violation and provide a time limit within which OSHA expects that the violation will be corrected.

It is important that you review the citation immediately. You might find that the time limit is not feasible, and you would want to contact the OSHA inspector to request more time. You must also post the citation in a prominent place in the affected area for a minimum of three days or until the violation is resolved. The sooner you can repair the problem and remove the violation, the better.

In addition to the citation, OSHA provides an assessment of the penalty along with instructions on how to either contest the penalty or pay the fine. Be sure to take the time to carefully review the OSHA citation and penalties assessed, not only to ensure that you understand them, but also to determine at what level you might actually be in compliance and whether you believe there is a discrepancy between your practices and what the violation alleges.

It is best to set up a settlement conference as soon as possible with the regional administrator of OSHA (see the "settlement conference" section later in this chapter for more information on whether to engage in such negotiations).

Penalty levels

OSHA assesses several violations and penalty levels. The maximum levels are as follows:

- Other than serious
- Serious violation
- Willful violation
- Repeat violation
- Failure to abate

Other than serious

This kind of violation deals with job safety and health not resulting in death or serious physical injury. The fine for such a violation may range from zero to $1,000 per violation.

OSHA could reduce the penalty for this violation by as much as 95% if the employer has demonstrated a good-faith effort, meaning the employer complies with OSHA regulations. OSHA could also reduce the fine if the facility has not had any previous violations, or if it did, they were minor in nature. Reductions could also come because of the size of the organization. Particularly in today's environment, OSHA is trying to be kinder to smaller and mid-sized businesses.

Serious violation

This violation concerns situations in which death or serious physical injury could occur. The fine for this violation, depending on the extent of the violation, ranges from $1,500 to $7,000 per violation.

Once again, OSHA could reduce the level of the penalty, based on the same principles mentioned previously, such as good faith, history, and size of the business.

Willful violation

This violation concerns a situation that the employer knows exists, and yet takes no action to correct. OSHA considers this to be one of the most serious violations. The fines associated with a willful violation are $70,000 per finding, although there is a minimum penalty of $5,000 OSHA could assess.

A willful violation could also lead to OSHA taking criminal action against an organization. The results are serious if there is a conviction. The OSHA penalty for an employer who is convicted in the death of an employee could be as high as $250,000 or $500,000 if the business is a corporation. Along with the monetary penalty is the possibility of imprisonment for up to six months. In addition, the law allows for doubling the imprisonment time if a second conviction occurs (*note:* This does not mean a second conviction for the same crime, but for a different crime of the same nature).

Repeat violation

A repeat violation refers to a violation of any OSHA regulation, rule, or order (a citation is an order) that, upon reinspection, still exists. It could also mean a similar violation that is comparable to, but not exactly like the first violation exists, which could result in a repeat violation citation. This type of violation typically occurs after the time that a previous citation has become a final order. In other words, the violation occurs after a settlement conference, or after a citation has been issued and posted and the time for correction has passed.

A repeat violation could occur up to three years after the initial finding. The resulting penalty could be as high as $70,000 per event. OSHA calculates the size of the penalty by adjusting the initial penalty for the size of the business, then multiplying that figure by two, five, or 10, depending on the size of the business.

Failure to abate

This violation refers to a citation that is given when a prior violation is not abated. This may result in penalties of up to $7,000 for each day the violation persists beyond the final abatement date.

Note that there is a difference between a repeat violation and a failure to abate. The former refers to a violation that has occurred within a three-year window, and the inspector comes back to review that matter and finds that it still exists. The latter citation is for a current violation that is not resolved in a timely fashion.

OSHA may issue citations and penalties under some other categories. These include

- falsifying records or reports, such as injury logs or monitoring data, which could result in fines of up to $10,000 per violation and/or six months in jail

- violations of posting requirements, such as a failure to post both the annual summary of injuries or illnesses and the safety and health rights of employees, which could result in fines of $7,000 per violation

- intimidating or interfering with a compliance officer in performance of his or her job, which could result in a fine of $5,000 and a jail sentence of up to three years

The settlement conference

The answer to whether you should seek a settlement conference is a resounding "yes." You or the administration should set up a settlement conference once you have had a chance to review the citation(s) and the penalties associated with the them, but certainly within the 15-day deadline for appeals or contest of the citation.

You should also take the time to review your institution's policies and procedures surrounding the particular violation, such as indoor air quality, ergonomics, or asbestos abatement. If OSHA finds you deficient in a policy or procedure, take the time and effort to fix the problem before you go to the settlement conference.

The settlement conference provides an opportunity for you to set the record straight and reduce the penalties leveled. You will not, in all likelihood, be able to eliminate all of the penalties assessed, but you might be able to substantially reduce them. The settlement conference will also give you and your organization an opportunity to develop a better relationship with the OSHA area director. You can show the area director that your organization's goals and OSHA's are most likely the same: providing a safe and healthful working environment for your employees. Developing this relationship will be helpful now and in the future.

Who should attend the conference?

One of the first questions that always arises when arranging a settlement conference, especially after a long and perhaps arduous inspection, is whether to bring your organization's lawyer. The answer to this question depends on how confrontational you wish to make the proceedings. Typically, settlement conferences are more informal in nature. Bringing a lawyer along will likely set the wrong tone for the meeting and the proceedings. You must, of course, use your own judgment, particularly if the violation is of the repeat nature. You can usually accomplish more without a lawyer present, although you should certainly review all of the information contained in the citation with your facility's attorneys prior to attending the conference.

Note that if you bring a lawyer, OSHA will likely bring one, too. If you do not bring a lawyer, OSHA will not likely bring one. However, like your organization's lawyers, OSHA's lawyers will have reviewed all of the information in advance.

When planning the conference, include the safety professional who took part in the tour, a representative from administration, and the department head in whose area or under whose responsibility the violation(s) occurred. For example, if there were problems with the policies and procedures for safe sharps devices and elimination of needlestick hazards, bring the infection control coordinator to the meeting. If the problem involved lockout/tagout procedures, include a representative from facilities maintenance at the conference.

Establish your agenda

Before attending the conference, be sure your organization's representatives are well versed in your position on the citations. Make sure they understand your organization's policies and procedures and what steps have been taken to address the violations. It is a reasonable expectation that that the inspector who conducted the inspection and cited you will join the area director in the conference.

Although the specific citations applied to your organization will dictate the conference's agenda, it is of critical importance that you present a reasoned approach to each of the cited areas. Failing to do so could result in the area director or the OSHA inspector leading the conversation, potentially causing you to make errors in your description of events or the circumstances surrounding the alleged violation. You must be an active participant in defense of your organization's policies and practices in order to counter OSHA's perceptions and interpretation of the alleged violations. Only in this way can you be sure that the OSHA representatives understand how your organization's compliance strategies were identified and implemented.

Explain that your decisions were based on logic and a rational process that considered compliance requirements as a function of providing the safest possible environment and that you had acted in the best interest of your facility. For example, if you were cited for violations of the needlestick prevention portion of the Bloodborne Pathogen standard because you were not using the most up-to-date prevention techniques or equipment available, demonstrate that your employees participated in the technology and equipment selection as prescribed by law. Explain that it was the decision of the line employees that newer equipment and technology was not warranted or necessary. This speaks volumes to the importance of documenting any and all compliance-related activities, from education sessions to product selection to safety rounds. These types of decisions should be documented in minutes of any meetings held on the topic. Be sure to take those minutes to the settlement conference.

Get the best possible results

The purpose of the settlement conference is to enable you to provide the OSHA representatives with a clear understanding of your organization's policies and positions and how those policies and positions result in your organization's compliance. You may elect to immediately challenge the findings of the inspector or even appeal them in writing within 15 days of the issuance of the citation and penalty.

However, at the settlement conference you have the opportunity to demonstrate that the inspector could have misinterpreted what he or she witnessed. For example, if there was no sign with the word "asbestos" on it warning of the presence of asbestos in a machine room, but only a sign with a colored stripe on it outside the door, the OSHA inspector could find it a violation of the "failure to warn" section of the hazard communication standard. However, if your safety officer can demonstrate that the facility has a policy indicating that a certain colored stripe on a sign warns of the presence of asbestos and that employees have been educated about this, then you can demonstrate that the inspector misinterpreted what he or she observed.

Use the settlement conference to show that you have either corrected the problem or are well on your way to doing so. Take this opportunity to reduce the monetary penalties to the lowest possible level. In addition, use this opportunity to establish good faith credit for future encounters. Both of these outcomes are in your institution's best interests and are the best possible results.

Conference review

Settlement conference proceedings may depend on how an area director asserts his or her own judgment within OSHA regulatory guidelines and on the quality of the relationship between your organization and the OSHA office. A good relationship naturally stands you in better stead than a contentious relationship.

The settlement conference typically begins with a review of the findings by the area director in collaboration with the inspector. You will be given an opportunity to describe the circumstances surrounding the alleged violations and why you think the citation should not stand. A discussion will ensue involving all parties. Ultimately, the decision is in the hands of the area director, who has the authority to propose a settlement that includes a reduction in the fine and a recommendation for the length of time he or she will allow you to correct the violation.

Many times, settlement conferences involve a number of citations. In that case, each one will be dealt with separately. At the conclusion of the settlement conference, OSHA personnel will redraft the citation, which an OSHA attorney must sign off on. Your organization will receive that final copy via the mail. Post the revised citation in a location where employees can view it.

Chapter

5

The relationship among regulators

The relationship among regulators

The JCAHO, EPA, and OSHA

OSHA does not exist in a vacuum. Other agencies, most notably the Joint Commission on Accreditation of Healthcare Organizations (JCAHO) and the Environmental Protection Agency (EPA), have crossover ties with OSHA and with one another. If one of these other agencies during an investigation observes a violation of an OSHA regulation, it could report it to OSHA. Even though the JCAHO has no authority to issue penalties or citations, it has an obligation, based on a written memorandum of understanding, to report OSHA violations.

The JCAHO

The JCAHO could make a report to OSHA for a variety of reasons. Although it may not always be obvious, the JCAHO, like OSHA, deals with safety issues, not only for patients, but also for workers. As mentioned earlier, while the JCAHO's charter results in a more patient-oriented focus, the JCAHO surveyors are sufficiently familiar with the most significant OSHA standards to be able to identify potential violations as the result of deficient practice.

The JCAHO's scrutiny of processes related to safety as a function of its accreditation process is of two-fold origin. The primary "driver" is the JCAHO's role in relation to the Centers for Medicare & Medicaid Services (CMS) Conditions of Participation. The Conditions of Participation outline the requirements that healthcare organizations must meet in order to participate in Medicare/Medicaid reimbursement, a key revenue stream for most healthcare organizations. Because the CMS has limited resources relative to ensuring that each of the participating healthcare organizations is in compliance with the Conditions of Participation, other organizations, most notably the JCAHO, have been given deemed status to conduct compliance surveys of organizations on behalf of the CMS.

Additionally, the JCAHO has ongoing relationships with many professional organizations, such as the National Fire Protection Association and the American Society of Safety Engineers, with whom the JCAHO has developed and implemented standards relating to safety, security, hazardous materials and waste, emergency management, life and fire safety, equipment management, and utilities management. Assessment of these functions, collectively known as the Environment of Care management standards, is a regular activity of the JCAHO accreditation survey process.

If during the course of a survey, especially during the tour of the physical plant, a JCAHO surveyor observes a failure on the part of the hospital to adequately protect employees from exposure to hazards, the surveyor may make a report to

OSHA, particularly if the JCAHO inspector feels that the situation is significant enough to cause harm to employees.

The JCAHO does not have the force of law behind it, as does OSHA. If a JCAHO surveyor sees repeated fire safety violations, such as blocked stairwells and locked fire exit doors, or a failure to monitor and record employee exposures to waste anesthetic gases, or unsafe handling and disposal of hazardous materials, these violations could prompt a call to OSHA, which has the power to impose penalties. That is not to say, however, that the JCAHO cannot exercise significant impact on your organization. A JCAHO survey finding can result in a denial of accreditation if the survey team determines that there is any circumstance that could result in a significant safety deficiency. The survey finding can also cite past practice, such as failing to adequately implement interim life safety measures, as a reason for accreditation restrictions. Also, noncompliance with any portion of the Conditions of Participation can result in grievous financial implications for your organization.

The EPA

The EPA and OSHA, as mentioned, also have cooperative agreements. For many years, the EPA did not conduct routine inspections of healthcare facilities. However, as discussed in the Chapter 1, the EPA has shown a new interest in healthcare organizations since the early 1990s.

The EPA's most recent forays into hospitals have concerned the issue of chemical waste storage and disposal as they relate to the Resource Conservation and Recovery Act (RCRA), which gives the EPA the authority to control hazardous waste inclusive of its transportation, treatment, storage, and disposal. RCRA also set forth a framework for the management of nonhazardous wastes.

During EPA inspections, if the inspectors observe egregious violations of worker safety, they can report these violations to OSHA. For example, asbestos removal from within the facility falls under OSHA's domain. However, when asbestos is released into the outdoor environment, EPA regulations like the National Emission Standards for Hazardous Air Pollutants (NESHAP) come into play. If the EPA inspector sees a NESHAP violation during the inspection, the inspector could also notify OSHA about it.

State-level OSHAs

In some states, a state-level OSHA replaces the federal OSHA. For a state to operate under its own OSHA and not under federal management, it must adopt regulations and requirements that are at least as stringent as those adopted and enforced at the federal level. California is one such example. Cal/OSHA is a strong leader in the promulgation and enforcement of workplace health and safety regulations, and has many regulations that exceed the federal OSHA standards.

Some states, such as Massachusetts, have both a federal OSHA and a state department of occupational health and safety. Typically in these circumstances, the requirements of both agencies are similar. One or the other, or in some cases both agencies could be called upon to investigate a complaint.

NIOSH

It is also important to mention the National Institute for Occupational Safety and Health (NIOSH), which at this writing, is under extreme governmental pressure to reorganize and to remove its direct reporting line from the head of the Centers for Disease Control and Prevention (CDC) to lower level personnel at the CDC. At the time of this writing, this has not yet occurred. However, reports in professional publications indicate that this restructuring of NIOSH and the CDC will occur soon.

The restructuring, it is feared, could affect the ability of NIOSH to obtain money and carry out its role in studying the health and safety aspects of a wide range of materials, such as the hazards of exposure to chemicals or examining the issues surrounding latex glove safety. There is also concern that these proposed changes could hurt NIOSH's ability to recommend and affect OSHA's decisions in crafting legislation for worker protection, ultimately weakening the entire system of worker protection in the United States.

NIOSH is not an enforcement arm of OSHA. It is a research and, occasionally, an investigative agent. Most often, NIOSH conducts research on various aspects of a proposed health and safety regulation, or will help through its work to define the limits of a safety device, such as respirators or safety goggles. In addition, employees may call upon NIOSH to come on-site and review a health and safety problem that they believe has gone unsolved. NIOSH investigators can collect data, interview employees, and make recommendations for the resolution of those problems.

Compliance is key

No matter which agency you work with, your key to a successful inspection is compliance. You must demonstrate to each organization that arrives at your facility that you are aware of, and proactively manage, employee health and safety, as well as environmental health and safety regulations. Establish that you are not only in current compliance, but that education and training will keep you compliant in the future.

With healthcare likely to remain one of the most regulated industries in the United States, OSHA is one of the most intimidating agencies in the mix of regulators. Over the past 15 to 20 years, OSHA has become more involved in healthcare worker safety, enacting and enforcing regulations in a wide range of topics from chemical safety to prevention of bloodborne diseases through exposure to contaminated needles. While absolute compliance and conformity to the regulations is always the best way to protect your institution, it may not always be realistic or practicable. Employee complaints, accidents, or worse yet, employee deaths occur in hospitals as in any other industry. Although employee deaths are infrequent events in healthcare, injuries and illnesses are not. Failure to appropriately manage efforts to minimize or eliminate such events may lead to an OSHA inspection.

OSHA inspections need not be disasters, nor should you think of them as the end of the line as a safety professional. Dealing with rules, regulations, and OSHA in a professional, competent, and educated way can only make your OSHA experience more positive and ensure the provision of a safe and healthful environment throughout your organization.